The Hearing Aid Handbook

Everything You Wish They Told You

David L. Etheridge

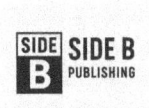

Side B Publishing

Copyright © 2025 by David Lawton Etheridge

All rights reserved.

No portion of this book may be reproduced in any form without written permission from the publisher or author, except as permitted by U.S. copyright law.

Contents

1. Dedication — 1
2. Note from the Author — 2
3. Welcome to the Club — 4
4. A Look Back — 6
5. Understanding Your Hearing Loss — 10
6. Meet Your Ears — 16
7. Getting to Know Your Device — 20
8. Understanding Costs and Options — 25
9. The First Few Weeks — 28
10. Mastering Your Hearing Aids — 32
11. Living Your Life with Hearing Aids — 36
12. Tips from Longtime Users — 41
13. Final Thoughts — 43
14. About the Author — 46
15. Hearing Aid Glossary — 48
16. Troubleshooting Quick-Reference — 51
17. Resources — 57
18. Thank You — 58

Dedication

To my dad

The man who introduced me to this world, walked beside me in it, and taught me how to lead with integrity, empathy, and grace. Thank you for the opportunity to build a life beside you—as a son, a business partner, and a man. Those years were more than a career. They were a gift. This book, and the heart behind it, exists because of you.

And to my mom

Who cheered us on, kept us grounded, and stepped in as referee when needed (more than once). You showed me the meaning of unconditional support, and saw the best in both of us even when we couldn't. Thanks for holding everything together with kindness, faith, humor, and a whole lot of love.

Note from the Author

I didn't set out to write a book. I just knew that if I ever did, it had to be something that meant something. And this—helping people reconnect with their world through better hearing—means a lot to me.

I spent over a decade in the hearing aid industry, working alongside my dad in a franchise we co-owned and operated together. We worked hard, treated people right, and did our best to make a difference. It wasn't glamorous. It wasn't always easy. But it mattered. We helped people hear again—and I got to do that with someone who had spent his life helping me find my own voice.

This book isn't about selling hearing aids. It's about helping you *use* them. It's about the honest, often awkward, occasionally hilarious process of learning to hear again—and knowing you're not alone while you do it.

I may have left the hearing aid business, but all those years of learning what worked, what didn't, and how to truly support people through this journey—that knowledge stayed with me. I didn't want it to just sit unused or get lost to time, so I put it here, hoping it might reach someone who needs it.

The tools will change. The technology will change. And maybe someday, this book won't be needed. But if today it helps you take even one step forward with a little more confidence, then I'll be grateful I wrote it.

This book is for anyone starting—or restarting—their hearing aid journey. Whether you're a first-time user looking for clarity, a family member eager to support someone you care about, or someone revisiting hearing aids after a less-than-perfect experience, these pages were written with you in mind.

If you're holding this book, chances are you or someone you love is at the beginning of this journey. My hope is that these pages make the path smoother—offering reassurance when things sound strange, and reasons to celebrate as the world starts sounding sweet again.

Thanks for letting me be a small part of your journey.

~David L. Etheridge

Welcome to the Club

It's Not as Scary as You Think

Welcome to the hearing aid club—a place nobody really wants to join, but where you'll find you're in surprisingly good company.

Maybe you're feeling hopeful about your new hearing aids. Maybe you're overwhelmed. Or maybe—if we're being honest—you're wondering what you've just gotten yourself into. If that sounds familiar, take a deep breath. Every club member I've met has felt exactly what you're feeling right now.

This chapter is all about normalizing the experience of starting your hearing aid journey. While no two stories are exactly the same, there are some pretty universal emotions that come up: relief, frustration, surprise, and even joy. Yes, joy. That moment when you hear birds chirping again for the first time? It's real. And it's powerful.

But let's not sugarcoat things—there's an adjustment period. Things will sound different. Your brain will have to relearn how to interpret certain sounds. You might get tired of wearing them by the end of the day. You might even be tempted to toss them in a drawer and forget the whole thing. (Spoiler alert: don't do that.)

This is a process. And like any process, it comes with good days and tough ones. The key is patience—with the devices, with your brain, and with yourself. Your hearing didn't change overnight, and neither will your experience of sound.

So what does this adjustment period actually look like? Let me give you the real picture—both the challenges and the victories.

Here's what you can expect:

- Sounds that seem "too loud" or "tinny" at first

- Your own voice sounding strange (we call that the occlusion effect)

- Fatigue from processing new levels of sound

- The occasional itch or discomfort as your ears adjust

And here's what else you can expect:

- Gradual improvement as your brain adapts

- Clearer conversations with friends and family

- Less strain in noisy places (once you learn some tricks—more on that later)

- A boost in confidence when you realize you're not missing out anymore

In these pages, you'll find the tricks nobody told you at your fitting, the honest answers to questions you didn't know to ask, and maybe even a few laughs along the way. Think of me as your club sponsor—someone who's been here before and wants to help you navigate the experience with a little more confidence and a lot less confusion.

So welcome to the club. You've taken a big step, and that deserves some credit. Let's get started.

A Look Back

From Ear Trumpets to Smartphones: Why Today's Hearing Aids Are Nothing Like Your Grandfather's

If you're hesitant about hearing aids because you picture those flesh-colored chunks your grandmother wore, or you're worried about looking "old" with something hanging off your ear, let me paint you a different picture. The hearing aids available today are so far removed from what previous generations used that they're barely the same category of device.

Understanding this evolution isn't just a history lesson—it's about recognizing that you're living in the golden age of hearing technology.

The Humble (and Embarrassing) Beginnings

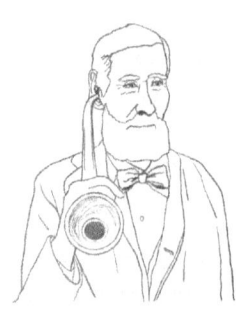

Picture this: It's 1650, and you're struggling to hear conversations. Your solution? A three-foot-long metal horn that you hold up to your ear while pointing the wide end at whoever's speaking. These ear trumpets were about as subtle as a megaphone and roughly as portable as a fishing pole.

The wealthy tried to make them fashionable—decorating them with engravings or disguising them as fans. But there was no hiding the fact that hearing help meant carrying around what essentially amounted to a small tuba. Despite the awkwardness, people used them because the alternative was isolation.

When Electricity Changed Everything (Sort Of)

Alexander Graham Bell's invention of the telephone in the 1870s accidentally solved a hearing problem. His carbon microphone could amplify sound electrically—a breakthrough that wasn't lost on Bell, whose mother and wife both had hearing loss.

But here's what those early "electric" hearing aids looked like: imagine a desk-sized radio with wires running to headphones. Users had to sit at a table, plug into the wall, and hope whoever they wanted to talk to would stay put long enough for a conversation. Not exactly conducive to a social life.

The 1920s brought vacuum tubes, which shrank hearing aids down to the size of a cigarette pack. Progress! Except now you wore a box clipped to your belt with wires running up to your ears under your clothes. Better than the desk model, but still obvious to anyone paying attention.

The Breakthrough That Changed Everything

The transistor revolution of the 1950s was the game-changer. Suddenly, hearing aids could fit behind your ear instead of in your pocket. They were still visible, still obviously "hearing aids," but for the first time, they weren't announcing themselves from across the room.

This was also when audiologists started understanding that different people needed different kinds of help. Instead of just "making everything louder," hearing aids began targeting specific frequency ranges where individuals had the most trouble.

The Digital Revolution: Your Hearing Aids Get Smart

The 1990s brought digital processing, and this is where hearing aids stopped being simple amplifiers and became sophisticated computers. For the first time, your hearing aids could:

- Distinguish between speech and background noise
- Automatically adjust to different environments
- Remember your preferences for different situations
- Provide precise amplification only where you needed it

This was revolutionary because it solved the biggest complaint people had about hearing aids: "Everything is too loud!" Digital processing meant your hearing aids could make voices clearer without turning the lawn mower into a jet engine.

Today: The Technology Your Grandparents Could Never Imagine

Modern hearing aids are essentially tiny computers that happen to help you hear better. They can:

- Stream phone calls directly to your ears (no more fumbling with the phone)
- Play music wirelessly from your smartphone
- Adjust automatically when you walk from a quiet room into a restaurant
- Reduce wind noise when you're outside
- Enhance speech clarity in noisy environments
- Track your physical activity and even detect falls
- Be controlled entirely from an app on your phone[1]
- Recharge overnight like your smartphone (no more tiny batteries)

Some are completely invisible when worn. Others are so small they're barely noticeable. And the sound quality? It's often better than what people with normal hearing experience naturally.

What This Means for You Right Now

Here's why this history matters: every concern you might have about hearing aids—they're too visible, they make everything too loud, they're inconvenient, they mark you as "old"—has been solved by modern technology.

Your great-grandfather would have given anything for what you can slip discretely into your ears today. Where he dealt with bulky, obvious devices that barely worked, you have access to nearly invisible computers that can be fine-tuned to your exact hearing loss and lifestyle.

The stigma around hearing aids largely comes from outdated mental images of what they used to be. But if you've seen someone wearing modern hearing aids and didn't even notice them, that tells you everything you need to know about how far we've come.

The Bottom Line

You're not choosing between hearing well and looking good—that trade-off disappeared years ago. You're choosing between staying connected to the world around you and gradually missing more of life's important moments.

The people who came before you made do with ear trumpets and tabletop amplifiers because they understood something crucial: staying engaged with family, friends, and the world around them was worth whatever inconvenience the technology required.

You get to make the same choice, but with technology that would seem like magic to previous generations. The question isn't whether today's hearing aids are good enough—it's whether you're ready to take advantage of just how good they've become.

Now that you understand you're working with 21st-century technology, not your grandfather's hearing aids, let's talk about how that technology gets customized specifically for your hearing needs.

Let's take a closer look at why you needed those tools in the first place—starting with your hearing test and what it really tells you.

---

[1] National Institute on Deafness and Other Communication Disorders (NIDCD). *Hearing Aids*. Updated March 2023. https://www.nidcd.nih.gov/health/hearing-aids

Understanding Your Hearing Loss

What the Test Reveals

Making Sense of Your Hearing Test

You walk out of the audiologist's office with a piece of paper covered in dots, lines, and numbers. The professional who tested you rattled off some terms and percentages, but honestly? You're not entirely sure what any of it means for your day-to-day life.

If this sounds familiar, you're not alone. Most people leave their hearing test with more questions than answers. But here's the thing: that piece of paper in your hand is actually a detailed blueprint of how you hear the world—and understanding it puts you in the driver's seat of your hearing health journey.

What Actually Happened During Your Test

Let's start with what you just experienced. That hearing test (called an audiogram) wasn't just random beeping—it was systematically mapping how your ears respond to different sounds.

The pure tone testing, where you raised your hand or pressed a button when you heard beeps, was checking the quietest sounds you can detect at various pitches. Think of it like testing the sensitivity of a radio across different stations.

When they had you repeat words back, they were measuring something entirely different: how well your brain processes speech once it reaches your ears. You might hear the sound clearly but still struggle to understand what was said—and this test reveals that gap.

The bone conduction test, where they placed that vibrating device behind your ear, was essentially giving your hearing a "back door" entrance. By bypassing your outer and middle ear entirely, it shows whether the problem lies in the mechanics of getting sound to your inner ear, or in your inner ear itself.

Decoding Your Personal Hearing Map

Now, about that chart. Imagine your audiogram as a topographical map of your hearing landscape. The horizontal axis shows pitch (frequency)—from the low rumble of thunder on the left to the high chirp of a smoke detector on the right. The vertical axis shows volume (intensity)—from whisper-quiet at the top to rock-concert-loud at the bottom.

Every dot on your chart represents the softest sound you could hear at that particular pitch. The lower the dot sits on the chart, the louder that sound had to be before you could detect it.

Here's what matters most: the zone between 250 and 6000 Hz is where most human speech lives. The consonants that help you distinguish between "cat" and "bat," the subtle inflections that tell you whether someone is asking a question or making a statement—it all happens in this critical frequency range.

Your hearing loss level tells a story about your daily experience:

Mild hearing loss (26-40 dB) means you're missing the subtle sounds—whispers, distant conversations, the soft footsteps of someone approaching. You probably find yourself asking "What?" more often, especially in quiet settings.

Moderate hearing loss (41-55 dB) makes regular conversation challenging, particularly when there's background noise. You might notice you're reading lips more, or that phone conversations have become frustrating.

Severe hearing loss (71-90 dB) means you're likely hearing only the loudest environmental sounds and voices. Conversations without visual cues become nearly impossible.

Profound hearing loss (91+ dB) shifts your communication style significantly—you might rely heavily on visual cues, lip reading, or feeling vibrations.

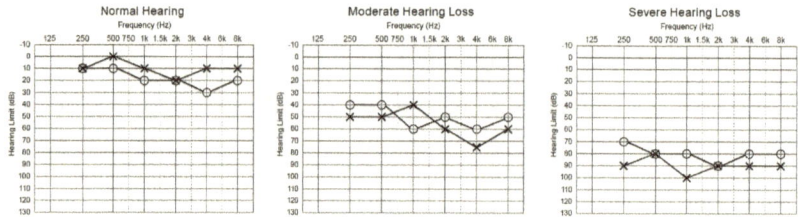

Normal, Moderate, and Severe Test Result Examples on an Audiogram

I know—charts and decibels aren't everyone's thing. But once you get this, you'll start seeing what your ears *can* and *can't* do—and how to help them out.

The Three Types of Hearing Loss (And Why It Matters)

Your hearing loss also has a "type" that affects your treatment options:

Conductive hearing loss means something is blocking or interfering with sound getting to your inner ear—maybe earwax, fluid, or a structural issue. The good news? This type is often medically treatable.

Sensorineural hearing loss involves damage to your inner ear or the nerve pathways to your brain. This is the most common type and usually results from aging, noise exposure, or genetics. While typically permanent, it responds well to hearing aids.

Mixed hearing loss combines both types, which means you might benefit from medical treatment and hearing aids.

Why This All Matters for Your Next Steps

If you decide to explore hearing aids, your audiogram becomes their programming guide. Modern hearing aids don't just "turn up the volume"—they're sophisticated computers that can amplify the exact frequencies where you need help while leaving your good hearing alone.

Think of it this way: if your hearing loss mainly affects high frequencies, your hearing aids will boost those cricket chirps and consonant sounds while leaving the low-frequency rumble of traffic relatively untouched. This precision is why two people with hearing aids might have completely different experiences—their devices are tuned to their unique hearing fingerprint.

Your Next Move

Understanding your hearing test results isn't just academic—it's practical power. When you meet with hearing care professionals, you can ask specific questions: "I see my hearing drops off significantly at 4000 Hz—how will that affect my ability to hear my grandchildren?" or "My speech understanding scores were lower in my left ear—will that influence which hearing aid features I need?"

Don't let anyone brush past the explanation with technical jargon. This is your hearing, your daily experience, and your decision. The more you understand about your specific hearing profile, the more confident you'll feel about whatever path you choose—whether that's hearing aids, medical treatment, or simply monitoring your hearing over time.

Ready to Take Action? Your Step-by-Step Guide

If you're feeling motivated to move forward but aren't sure how, here's a practical roadmap:

Step 1: Book Your Hearing Evaluation

Start with your primary care doctor if you prefer, or go straight to a hearing care professional. Look for these credentials: Au.D. (Doctor of Audiology), NBC-HIS (National Board Certified Hearing Instrument Specialist), or state-licensed professionals.

Before booking, ask whether the hearing test is free, covered by your insurance, or included in a consultation fee. Many providers offer complimentary evaluations.

Step 2: Choose Your Care Style

Consider what type of ongoing relationship you want:

Private clinics typically offer more personalized care, longer appointments, and comprehensive follow-up. You'll likely see the same person each visit and get more hand-holding through the adjustment process.

Big-box stores often have competitive pricing and decent technology, but less customization and shorter appointment times. Good for straightforward hearing loss and budget-conscious buyers.

Online/mail-in options offer convenience and lower costs, but limited hands-on support. Best for tech-savvy individuals comfortable with self-adjustment.

Choose based on your comfort level, budget, and how much guidance you want throughout the process.

Step 3: Ask the Right Questions

Come prepared with questions that matter to you:

- What specific type of hearing loss do I have, and how might it progress?
- Which hearing aid styles would work best for my lifestyle and dexterity?
- What's included in the total cost? (Follow-up visits, adjustments, warranties, accessories)
- What's your trial period and return policy?
- What should I realistically expect during the first month of wearing hearing aids?

Step 4: Give Yourself Permission to Go Slow

You don't need to make any decisions on the spot. Take time to process the information, discuss it with family, or even seek a second opinion. This is a significant decision about your quality of life—you deserve to feel completely confident about your choice.

Remember: taking the first step to understand your hearing doesn't commit you to anything except becoming more informed about your own health. And that's always a win.

Next up, let's get better acquainted with the star of the show: your ears.

Meet Your Ears

Anatomy and Audiology Made Simple

Your ears are amazing. They're small, but they're responsible for helping you communicate, stay balanced, and enjoy everything from your favorite music to the laughter of loved ones. If you're going to wear hearing aids, it's helpful to understand what they're working with. Think of your ears as a sophisticated sound processing system with three main stages, each with a specific job. When you understand how this system works, choosing and adjusting to hearing aids becomes much clearer.

Stage 1: The Outer Ear - Your Sound Collector

The visible part of your ear—that curved structure on the side of your head—is called the auricle, or pinna. Its unique shape isn't just for looks. Those ridges and curves work like a satellite dish, capturing sound waves from different directions and funneling them into your ear canal.

Your ear canal does more than just carry sound inward. It naturally amplifies certain frequencies, particularly those in the range of human speech. This built-in amplification is one reason why a blocked ear canal from earwax can make everything sound muffled.

Stage 2: The Middle Ear - Your Sound Amplifier

Behind your eardrum lies a small, air-filled chamber containing three tiny bones with memorable names: the hammer (malleus), anvil (incus), and stirrup (stapes). These bones, collectively called ossicles, create a lever system that amplifies sound vibrations by about 20 times before passing them to the inner ear.

This amplification system is crucial because sound must transition from traveling through air to traveling through the fluid-filled inner ear. Without this mechanical boost, most sounds would be too weak to register.

When you have a cold or ear infection, fluid can fill this middle ear space, preventing the bones from moving freely. This is why everything sounds dim and distant when you're congested—the amplifier isn't working properly.

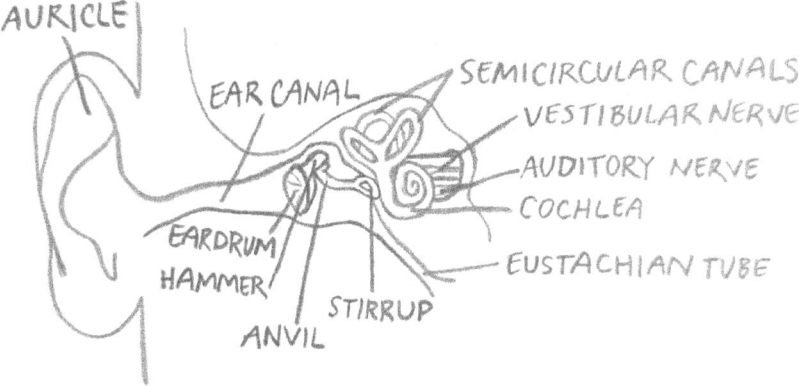

Stage 3: The Inner Ear - Your Sound Translator

The inner ear contains the cochlea, a snail-shaped structure about the size of a pea. Inside this spiral chamber, thousands of microscopic hair cells are arranged like piano keys, each tuned to respond to specific frequencies. High-frequency sounds trigger hair cells at the base of the cochlea, while low frequencies activate cells near the top.

When these hair cells detect vibrations, they convert the mechanical energy into electrical signals that travel along the auditory nerve to your brain. This is where most permanent hearing loss occurs. Unlike other cells in your body, these hair cells cannot regenerate once damaged by aging, noise exposure, medications, or genetics.

Your Brain: The Real Hearing Center

Here's a crucial insight: your ears don't actually "hear" anything. They collect and process sound, but your brain does the interpreting. Your brain recognizes patterns, filters out background noise, and gives meaning to the electrical signals it receives.

This is why two people with identical hearing test results can have very different experiences. One person's brain might excel at filling in missing speech sounds, while another struggles to understand conversations in noisy environments.

Understanding this brain-ear partnership explains why adjusting to hearing aids often requires patience. Your brain needs time to relearn how to process sounds it hasn't heard clearly in months or years.

What This Means for Your Hearing Aid Journey

Knowing where your hearing loss originates helps determine the best treatment approach:

Conductive hearing loss occurs when sound can't reach the inner ear effectively, often due to earwax buildup, fluid, or problems with the eardrum or middle ear bones. This type of hearing loss can sometimes be medically or surgically corrected.

Sensorineural hearing loss happens when hair cells in the inner ear are damaged. This is the most common type of permanent hearing loss and typically requires hearing aids programmed to compensate for the specific frequencies you can no longer hear naturally.

Mixed hearing loss combines both types and requires a comprehensive approach to treatment.

Your hearing care provider uses detailed testing to map exactly which frequencies are affected and by how much. This creates a blueprint for programming hearing aids that will provide the right amount of amplification where you need it most, without over-amplifying sounds you can already hear well.

Building Your Foundation

Think of this ear anatomy knowledge as the foundation for everything else you'll learn about hearing aids. When you understand how your natural hearing system works, you'll better appreciate how hearing aids can step in to help where your ears need support.

In the next chapter, we'll explore how hearing aids are designed to work with your ear's natural processes, examining their components and how they can be customized to your unique hearing profile.

Getting to Know Your Device

What Each Part Does

Understanding Modern Hearing Aids: A Complete Guide

Modern hearing aids are remarkable pieces of technology that transform how millions of people experience sound. Despite their small size, these devices contain sophisticated components working together to provide clear, personalized hearing assistance. Whether you're considering hearing aids for yourself or a loved one, understanding how they work will help you make informed decisions and get the most from your investment.

The Three Main Types of Hearing Aids

Before diving into components, it's helpful to understand the three primary styles available today:

Behind-the-Ear (BTE) models sit comfortably behind your ear with tubing that connects to an earmold or dome inside your ear canal. These offer the most power and are suitable for all levels of hearing loss.

In-the-Ear (ITE) devices fit entirely within your outer ear, making them less visible while still providing easy access to controls.

Receiver-in-Canal (RIC) hearing aids combine the best of both worlds—the main body sits behind your ear like a BTE, but the speaker (receiver) is placed directly in your ear canal for more natural sound quality.

How Hearing Aids Process Sound

Think of your hearing aid as a sophisticated audio processing system that works in real-time to enhance your hearing experience. Here's how sound travels through the device:

Step 1: Sound Collection

The process begins with **microphones**—small openings typically located on the top or front of the device. Modern hearing aids use dual microphones that work together like your natural ears do. These microphones don't just passively collect sound; they actively analyze your environment to distinguish between speech you want to hear and background noise you don't.

Step 2: Digital Processing

Once sound enters the microphones, it travels to the **amplifier**—essentially a miniature computer that performs millions of calculations per second. This digital processor is where the real magic happens. It can identify different types of sounds (speech, music, wind noise), adjust volume levels for different frequencies, and even predict what you want to hear based on your listening environment.

The amplifier doesn't simply make everything louder. Instead, it provides precise adjustments based on your specific hearing loss pattern. For example, if you have trouble hearing high-pitched sounds but can hear low-pitched sounds well, the amplifier will boost only the frequencies you need while leaving others unchanged.

Step 3: Sound Delivery

After processing, the refined sound travels to the **receiver** (also called the speaker). This tiny component converts the digital signal back into sound waves and delivers them directly into your ear. In RIC models, the receiver sits right in your ear canal for the most natural sound quality possible.

Power and Control Features

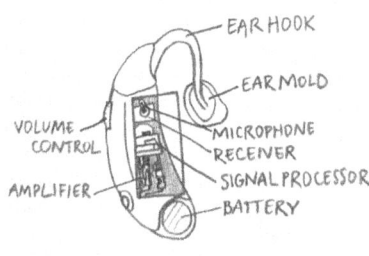

Battery Technology has evolved significantly in recent years. Traditional zinc-air batteries provide reliable power for 3-7 days depending on usage, while newer rechargeable lithium-ion batteries offer all-day power with overnight charging. Many users prefer rechargeable options because they eliminate the need to handle tiny batteries and reduce long-term costs.

Control Options have become increasingly sophisticated and user-friendly. While some hearing aids still include physical buttons for volume and program changes, many now connect to smartphone apps that provide intuitive control over every aspect of your hearing experience. These apps often include features like remote fine-tuning by your hearing care provider, GPS-based automatic program switching, and even translation services.

Comfort and Fit Components

Domes and Earmolds serve as the critical interface between your hearing aid and your ear. Domes are small, soft silicone pieces that come in various shapes (open, closed, or power) and sizes to match your ear canal and hearing needs. Custom earmolds are precisely crafted from impressions of your ears, providing the most secure fit and preventing feedback for people with severe hearing loss.

Wax Management Systems protect your investment and ensure consistent performance. Your ears naturally produce wax, which is healthy and normal, but it can interfere with hearing aid function if it blocks the receiver. Modern hearing aids include replaceable wax guards or filters that catch debris before it causes problems. Learning to replace these simple components can prevent many common issues.

Specialized Components for Different Styles

BTE Connectivity relies on tubing and hooks to connect the main device to your earmold. This tubing is designed to be flexible and durable, but it may need replacement over time as it can harden or develop cracks. Regular inspection of tubing ensures optimal sound quality and comfort.

Advanced Features in Modern Hearing Aids

Today's hearing aids often include cutting-edge features that were unimaginable just a few years ago. Many models offer Bluetooth connectivity for direct streaming from phones, televisions, and other devices. Some include artificial intelligence that learns your preferences and automatically adjusts settings based on your listening history. Advanced noise reduction algorithms can separate speech from background noise with remarkable precision, while directional microphones can focus on conversations happening directly in front of you.

The Benefits of Understanding Your Device

Knowledge about your hearing aid's components empowers you to take better care of your device, communicate more effectively with your hearing care provider, and troubleshoot minor issues independently. When you understand how each part functions, you can better articulate concerns during appointments, make informed decisions about upgrades or replacements, and feel more confident in your daily hearing aid use.

Understanding your hearing aid also helps you recognize when something isn't working properly. Is the sound distorted? Check your wax guard. Is the volume inconsistent? Your battery might need replacement or charging. Has the sound quality changed? Your tubing might need inspection.

Conclusion

Modern hearing aids represent a remarkable convergence of acoustic engineering, computer science, and user-centered design. By understanding how these components work together, you're better equipped to maximize your hearing aid's potential and maintain your connection to the sounds that matter most in your life. Whether you're navigating a busy restaurant, enjoying music, or having an intimate conversation, your hearing aids are working continuously to provide the clearest, most natural hearing experience possible.

Now let's talk about costs.

Understanding Costs and Options

Let's talk about the elephant in the room: hearing aids aren't cheap.

If you've been shocked by hearing aid prices, you're in good company. The cost can feel overwhelming, especially when you're already dealing with hearing challenges. This chapter breaks down what you're actually paying for and how to navigate your options without breaking the bank.

So... how much do hearing aids cost?

Hearing aids typically cost **$1,000 to $7,000 for a pair**[2], with most people spending around **$3,000 to $5,000** total. But here's what many people don't realize: that price isn't just for two small devices.

When you purchase hearing aids, you're paying for a complete care package that includes:

Professional Services: Your audiologist will test your hearing, program the devices specifically for your hearing loss, and fine-tune them as you adjust. This personalized fitting is crucial—hearing aids aren't one-size-fits-all.

Ongoing Support: Most providers include follow-up appointments, adjustments, cleaning, and maintenance for at least the first year. Think of it like buying a car with service included.

Protection: Warranties typically cover repairs and replacements for loss or damage, which matters when you're wearing $3,000+ devices daily.

Insurance Reality Check

Unfortunately, most insurance doesn't help much with hearing aids. Traditional Medicare doesn't cover them at all[3]. Some Medicare Advantage plans offer partial coverage, and a few private insurance plans might cover hearing tests but rarely the aids themselves.

Veterans have better options through the VA, and some state programs offer assistance for those who qualify financially.

Are there more affordable options?

Yes—there are now more options than ever. The hearing aid landscape has changed dramatically in recent years. Over-the-counter options now exist for mild to moderate hearing loss, starting around $200 to $1,500 per pair. Online retailers and big-box stores have entered the market with competitive pricing.

However, if you have complex hearing loss, struggle with small buttons and controls, or want personalized professional support, the traditional audiology route often provides better long-term results despite the higher upfront cost.

Can I try them first?

Yes—and you should. Never buy hearing aids without a trial period. Reputable providers offer 30 to 60 days to test the devices in your real life, with full refunds if they don't work for you. This trial period isn't optional—it's essential. Your hearing needs are unique, and what works for others might not work for you.

Ask before you buy. If they don't offer a trial, consider looking elsewhere.

Bottom Line:

Hearing aids are expensive, but consider the cost of not hearing well: missed conversations, safety concerns, social isolation, and potential cognitive impacts. The key is finding the right balance between your budget, your hearing needs, and the level of professional support that makes sense for your situation.

Start by getting a comprehensive hearing test, ask detailed questions about what's included in the price, and don't rush the decision. Your hearing health is worth the investment in research and careful consideration.

Coming up next: how to actually *adjust* to your new devices—and what nobody tells you about those first few weeks.

---

[2] Consumer Affairs. *Hearing aid costs in 2024.* https://www.consumeraffairs.com/health/hearing-aids-cost.html

[3] Medicare.gov. *Hearing aids & exams.* https://www.medicare.gov/coverage/hearing-aids

The First Few Weeks
What No One Tells You

The first few weeks with hearing aids aren't about getting everything perfect—they're about giving your brain time to remember how to hear again. Think of it like physical therapy for your ears. You wouldn't expect to run a marathon after knee surgery, and you shouldn't expect perfect hearing on day one either.

Week 1: Everything Feels Different (And That's Normal)

Your world just got louder. Paper crinkles like thunder. Footsteps sound like elephants. Your own chewing might make you wince. This isn't a sign something's wrong—it's proof something's right. Your brain had been turning down the volume on these sounds for months or years. Now it's getting the full soundtrack again.

Your voice sounds weird. Many people describe it as echoey or booming. This "occlusion effect" happens because your ear canal is now partially blocked. Your brain will adapt, and your audiologist can adjust the fit if it's really bothering you.

You'll feel tired. Listening is work, especially when your brain is processing sounds it hasn't heard clearly in ages. Mental fatigue is completely normal. Take breaks when you need them, but try to wear your aids a little longer each day.

Week 2-3: The Emotional Rollercoaster

Don't be surprised if you get teary hearing birds sing or your grandchild's laugh. Restored hearing can trigger powerful emotions—joy, grief for what you missed, even frustration when things still don't sound "right." All of these feelings are part of the process.

You might also feel self-conscious. Will people stare? Will they treat you differently? Here's the reality: most people either don't notice or don't care. And those who do comment are usually supportive or curious, not judgmental.

Your Daily Adjustment Toolkit

Instead of constantly fiddling with volume or switching programs, try these targeted exercises for 15-30 minutes daily:

Sound Mapping: Turn your faucet on and off, open and close cabinet doors. Sit in different spots while watching TV. These simple changes help your brain build a map of how sound works in your space.

The Three-Sound Challenge: Each day, identify three specific sounds—maybe the hum of your refrigerator, birds outside, or distant traffic. Focus on each one for a few minutes. Notice how they change throughout the day.

Phone Practice: Call someone you're comfortable with for short conversations. Phone audio is notoriously tricky with hearing aids, so regular practice builds confidence.

Subtitle Weaning: Start with familiar shows and gradually turn off captions. Don't stress if you miss things—this is training, not a test.

Public Places Practice: Visit a coffee shop or grocery store and pick one sound to follow—maybe a conversation at the next table or the espresso machine. Don't try to hear everything; just practice focusing on one audio source while filtering out the rest.

Directional Listening: Ask a friend or partner to speak while facing away from you, then toward you. Can you still understand them? This back-and-forth practice strengthens your ability to use visual cues and directional hearing together.

Consistency is key—try to spend at least 15–30 minutes a day doing something that helps your ears and brain work together.

When to Call Your Audiologist

Your initial fitting is just the starting point. Schedule follow-up appointments and come prepared with specifics:

- "Voices sound muffled during family dinners"
- "I hear a whistling sound when I hug people"
- "Everything sounds tinny in my car"

The more specific you are, the better they can help.

Ready to tackle some of the trickier stuff next? Let's get into feedback, volume issues, and that classic nemesis: background noise.. Stick with it, stay curious, and don't be afraid to ask for help. And remember, you're building a new relationship with sound—and like any relationship, it takes time.

> ### If You've Tried Before and Gave Up
>
> Maybe this isn't your first rodeo. If your hearing aids ended up in a drawer, you're not alone—and you're not crazy for being hesitant to try again. The truth is, adjusting takes time, and if no one guided you through it, of course it felt like a waste of time and money.
>
> Hearing aids have come a long way in recent years. The technology is better, sure—but more importantly, we've learned a lot about how people actually adjust to using them. And most people don't adjust overnight. The learning curve is real. The frustrations are real. But I hope you will try again, because this time, you're walking in with more knowledge. With realistic expectations. With someone in your corner (even if it's just the pages of this book). And with a better sense of what you *should* expect from your provider, your devices, and yourself.
>
> If you give it another go, give yourself a little grace. You're not starting from scratch—you're starting from experience. And that's a powerful place to begin.

The Bottom Line

These first few weeks aren't about achieving perfect hearing—they're about building a new relationship with sound. Some days will be better than others. Some sounds will delight you; others might annoy you. That's all part of learning to hear again.

Be patient with yourself. Celebrate small victories. And remember: every day you wear your hearing aids is a day your brain gets stronger at processing sound. You're not just adjusting to a device—you're reclaiming a sense that connects you to the world around you.

That's worth a few weeks of weirdness.

Mastering Your Hearing Aids

Solutions for Common Challenges

Every hearing aid user encounters three main challenges: feedback whistling, volume problems, and background noise. Understanding these issues and knowing how to address them will transform your hearing experience from frustrating to confident.

Understanding and Stopping Feedback

Feedback creates that unmistakable high-pitched whistle when sound from your hearing aid's speaker loops back into its microphone. While annoying, feedback usually signals a simple, fixable problem.

Why feedback happens:

- Your hearing aid doesn't fit snugly in your ear
- Earwax or debris blocks the sound path
- Objects come too close to your hearing aid (phones, hands, hats, hugs)
- Your volume is set too high for your current fit

Quick fixes you can try:

1. Remove and reinsert your hearing aid, ensuring it sits properly

2. Check and clean your wax guard - replace if blocked

3. Lower your volume temporarily to see if whistling stops

4. Keep phones and hands at a slight distance from your ears

When to contact your provider: If feedback persists after trying these solutions, schedule an appointment. Your audiologist can adjust the fit, modify your hearing aid's feedback cancellation settings, or determine if you need new ear molds.

Solving Volume Problems

Volume issues rarely mean your hearing aids are broken - they usually indicate settings that need fine-tuning or temporary conditions affecting your hearing.

When everything sounds too loud:

- You might be in an unusually noisy environment that overwhelms your current settings
- Your brain may still be adjusting to hearing sounds you haven't heard clearly in years
- Check if you've accidentally activated a volume boost or specific program

Start by checking your hearing aid app or manually lowering the volume. If the problem persists across different environments, contact your audiologist for program adjustments.

When everything sounds too soft:

- Your battery might be running low
- Wax, lint, or moisture could be blocking your microphone or speaker
- Your hearing aid might have switched to an inappropriate program

Try replacing your battery first, then gently clean your hearing aid. Check your app to ensure you're using the right program for your current environment.

When volume seems right but clarity is wrong: Don't hesitate to describe exactly what you're experiencing. Tell your audiologist that "voices sound hollow," "music sounds tinny," or "everything echoes." These descriptions help them make precise adjustments to improve your sound quality.

Managing Background Noise

Background noise frustrates nearly every new hearing aid user because it's the most complex challenge to solve. Modern hearing aids significantly reduce background noise, but they can't eliminate it entirely.

Strategies You Can Use:

- Position yourself with your back to walls and face toward speakers

- Move closer to people you want to hear

- Use your hearing aid's directional microphone features (many activate automatically)

- Switch to your "restaurant" or "speech in noise" program in noisy environments

- Stream phone calls and music directly to your hearing aids to bypass background noise

Long-term improvement: Your brain needs time to relearn how to focus on important sounds while filtering out noise. This process, called auditory adaptation, improves significantly over 3-6 months of consistent hearing aid use.

Rather than avoiding noisy places, gradually expose yourself to challenging listening environments. Start with shorter periods and take breaks when you feel overwhelmed. Each exposure helps your brain become more efficient at processing sound.

The Learning Process

These challenges aren't signs that your hearing aids aren't working - they're normal parts of adjusting to better hearing. Each problem you solve builds your confidence and improves your overall experience.

Most issues resolve with minor adjustments, simple maintenance, or time for your brain to adapt. When problems persist, your audiologist has tools and expertise to help you find solutions.

Remember: successful hearing aid use is a skill that develops over time. Be patient with yourself as you learn, and don't hesitate to ask for help when you need it.

Next up, let's get out into the world and talk about how hearing aids fit into your daily life—work, play, and everything in between.

Living Your Life with Hearing Aids

Work, Play, and Relationships

You're Not Broken—You're Just Getting an Upgrade

Here's what nobody tells you about hearing aids: they don't just help you hear better—they help you live better. Yes, there's an adjustment period. Yes, some days will be harder than others. But once you find your rhythm, you'll discover that hearing aids aren't just medical devices—they're freedom devices.

Your New Superpowers (And How to Use Them)

At Work: Become the Person Who Actually Hears Everything

Remember those meetings where you smiled and nodded, hoping you caught the important parts? Those days are over. With hearing aids, you might actually become the most tuned-in person in the room. You'll notice office sounds you forgot existed—that colleague's persistent pen clicking, the hum of the air conditioning, even whispered side conversations. Don't worry, your brain will learn to filter out what doesn't matter.

Your action plan:

- Tell your coworkers about your hearing aids upfront. It removes any awkwardness if you need clarification.
- Claim the seat where you can see everyone's faces—expressions and lip reading

are powerful backup systems.

- Explore streaming features for phone calls and video conferences. Many hearing aids can connect directly to your devices.

At Home: Rediscovering Your Own Space

Your home is about to feel more alive. You'll hear your cat's footsteps, catch conversations from other rooms, and actually know when someone calls your name from upstairs. These aren't small changes—they're the building blocks of feeling present in your own life.

Your action plan:

- If your hearing aids can stream TV audio, use this feature liberally. Everyone wins when you're not asking for the volume to be cranked up.

- Set up different volume profiles for different times of day—quiet morning coffee versus lively dinner prep.

- Build hearing aid maintenance into your routine. A quick daily cleaning prevents the buildup of dust, cooking oils, and other home debris that can affect performance.

Social Situations: From Survival Mode to Enjoyment Mode

Restaurants and group gatherings used to be endurance tests. Now they can actually be fun again. The key is working with your hearing aids, not just wearing them.

Your strategy:

- Scout your seating like a pro. Avoid spots near kitchen doors, speakers, or high-traffic areas.

- Train your friends and family that "speak clearly" works better than "speak louder."

- Learn your hearing aid's different programs. Most have a "restaurant" or "noisy environment" setting that can be a game-changer.

The Relationship Factor

With Your Partner: Intimacy Isn't Just Physical

Hearing loss can create distance in relationships—not because anyone means for it to happen, but because connection relies on communication. Hearing aids can restore those quiet moments of connection: the soft laugh at a private joke, the whispered "I love you" before sleep, the ability to actually hear what your partner is saying from across the room.

Building connection:

- Have an honest conversation about what you need. Your partner isn't a mind reader.
- Find humor in the inevitable mishearings. Laughter builds intimacy.
- Face each other during important conversations. It's not just about hearing—it's about presence.

With Everyone Else: Setting the Ground Rules

The people in your life want to support you, but they need guidance. You're not asking them to change who they are—you're asking them to communicate in a way that works for both of you.

The conversation starters:

- "I'm adjusting to hearing aids, so if I ask you to repeat something, it's not about you—it's about me learning."
- "It helps when you face me while talking."
- "Could we turn down the background noise just a bit?"
- "If you see me looking confused, a gentle tap gets my attention better than raising your voice."

Most people appreciate the directness because it gives them a clear way to help.

Making It Work for Your Life

Here's the truth: hearing aids aren't one-size-fits-all, and your life shouldn't have to fit around them. Whether you're training for marathons and need sweat-resistant devices, traveling constantly and need long battery life, or just want to hear your grandchildren's stories without strain—your hearing aids should adapt to your lifestyle, not the other way around.

This is your life, amplified. Not changed, not limited—amplified.

When Things Get Tough (And They Sometimes Will)

Living with hearing aids isn't always smooth sailing. Some days the world will sound too loud, too tinny, or just wrong. Some conversations will still be hard to follow. Some people will still mumble or talk too fast or forget to face you.

That doesn't mean you're failing. It means you're human, living in a complex world with a sophisticated piece of technology that's helping you navigate it better than you could before.

On the hard days:

- Remember why you started this journey
- Reach out to your audiologist—they've heard every concern before
- Connect with others who wear hearing aids
- Give yourself credit for showing up and trying

Your Quick-Start Success Formula

If you take nothing else from this chapter, take this:

1. **Wear them every day.** Start with short periods if you need to, but be consistent. Your brain needs regular practice.

2. **Expect an adjustment period.** Things will sound strange at first. That's your

brain relearning how to hear, not a sign something's wrong.

3. **Keep your follow-up appointments.** Fine-tuning is where the magic happens. Be honest about what's working and what isn't.

4. **Communicate your needs clearly.** The people in your life want to help—give them specific ways to do it.

5. **Learn the maintenance basics.** Clean them, charge them, protect them. Good care extends their life and your satisfaction.

6. **Don't quit during the learning curve.** Most successful hearing aid users didn't love them immediately. They just didn't give up.

The Bottom Line

You're not broken, and you don't need to be "fixed." You're someone who's choosing to engage more fully with life, and hearing aids are one of your tools for doing exactly that. Some days will be better than others, but every day you wear them is a day you're investing in connection, presence, and the fullness of your own experience.

Your hearing aids don't define you—they free you to be more yourself.

Next up: Real stories from people who've been where you are now, complete with the wisdom, humor, and practical tips that only come from lived experience.

Tips from Longtime Users

Hacks, Habits, and Humor

Sometimes the best guidance comes not from experts or manuals, but from people who've walked the path before you. The voices in this chapter belong to seasoned hearing aid users who've agreed to share their hard-won wisdom—anonymously, but authentically. These aren't polished testimonials or marketing speak. They're real insights from real people who remember what it felt like to be where you are now.

Tip 1: The Break-In Period Is Real—Don't Judge Too Fast "I hated my first pair for the first two weeks. Then one morning, I realized I could hear the birds again. I've worn hearing aids for 12 years now, and I don't go anywhere without them."

Tip 2: Keep a Tiny Toolkit "A glasses case with a wax loop, a brush, extra batteries, and a cleaning cloth—that's my go-bag. If I don't have it, I feel like I'm forgetting my phone."

Tip 3: Own It "At first, I tried to hide them. Then I realized most people couldn't care less. Now, I show them off. I even got mine in bright red. People say, 'Cool hearing aids!' and I say, 'Right?'"

Tip 4: Don't Skip the Follow-Ups "Each appointment made my hearing better. My audiologist adjusted things I didn't even know could be changed. Now I actually look forward to the tune-ups."

Tip 5: Be Ready to Laugh "You're going to mishear stuff. Sometimes hilariously. Just last week, I thought someone asked if I wanted a 'lizard sandwich.' (They said, 'caesar salad.') Roll with it. It's part of the fun."

Tip 6: They're an Investment—Protect Them "I use a dehumidifier case every night and never leave mine in the car. I paid good money for these little guys—they get better treatment than my phone."

Tip 7: Learn the Tech at Your Own Pace "Bluetooth, apps, streaming—it's a lot. Pick one new thing at a time. Get good at that, then try the next feature. It's not a race."

Tip 8: You'll Be the One Giving Advice Soon "After a year, I found myself helping a friend adjust her new pair. It felt good. It reminded me how far I'd come."

Everyone's journey with hearing aids is unique, but these shared experiences reveal common threads: patience during the adjustment period, the importance of proper care, and the value of maintaining your sense of humor along the way. Success isn't measured by perfection—it's built through persistence, the right attitude, and the willingness to embrace both the challenges and the victories.

As you move forward on your own hearing aid journey, carry these voices with you. And remember, sooner than you think, you'll have your own stories to tell and wisdom to share with someone taking their first steps into better hearing.

Now let's wrap things up with a glossary and a go-to list of helpful resources for your journey ahead.

Final Thoughts

Your Hearing Journey Continues

Congratulations—you've completed this comprehensive guide to hearing aids and taken a significant step toward better hearing health. From understanding how your ears work to mastering troubleshooting techniques, you now have the knowledge and tools to navigate this journey with confidence.

But here's the truth: **this isn't a destination. It's a new beginning.**

Beyond the Adjustment Period

Wearing hearing aids isn't about flipping a switch to restore what you once had. It's about embracing a different way of experiencing sound—one that requires patience, practice, and yes, some courage. You're not just adapting to technology; you're learning to engage with the world in a new way.

Every conversation you join, every sound you rediscover, every moment you choose to stay present instead of withdrawing—these are victories worth celebrating. Some days will feel easier than others, and that's completely normal.

What Makes You Successful

The most successful hearing aid users share certain qualities, and you're already developing them:

Persistence: You understand that adjustment takes time and you're willing to work through challenges rather than give up.

Advocacy: You know your needs matter and you're learning to communicate them clearly to providers, family, and friends.

Curiosity: Instead of accepting "good enough," you ask questions and seek solutions when something doesn't feel right.

Realistic Expectations: You understand that hearing aids enhance your life significantly, even if they don't restore perfect hearing.

Your Ongoing Toolkit

Keep this book as your reference companion. Hearing aid technology evolves, your hearing may change, and new situations will arise. When they do, you'll have:

- **Troubleshooting skills** to handle common issues independently
- **Communication strategies** to navigate challenging listening environments
- **Technical knowledge** to work effectively with your hearing care provider
- **Confidence** to advocate for adjustments and improvements

A Final Reminder

Your hearing loss doesn't define you, but how you respond to it absolutely can. By choosing to address it actively—through hearing aids, communication strategies, and ongoing education—you're modeling something powerful for everyone around you.

You're showing that aging, health changes, and life's curveballs don't have to mean withdrawal or isolation. You're demonstrating that it's possible to adapt, learn, and continue engaging fully with life.

Moving Forward

Stay curious about new developments in hearing technology. Keep practicing the communication strategies you've learned. Don't hesitate to schedule follow-up appointments when something doesn't feel right. And remember: every question you ask makes you a more informed and successful hearing aid user.

Most importantly, be patient with yourself. Some days your hearing aids will feel like a seamless part of you. Other days, you'll be more aware of them. Both experiences are normal parts of this ongoing journey.

Your hearing story doesn't end here—it evolves with you.

Here's to reconnecting with the sounds that matter most, the conversations that bring you joy, and the confidence that comes from taking control of your hearing health.

Welcome to your new chapter. It's going to be a good one.

About the Author

I spent over a decade working in the hearing aid industry, certified by the American Conference of Audioprosthology (ACA) and formerly by the National Board for Certification in Hearing Instrument Sciences (NBC-HIS). I also served as Secretary on the North Carolina Association of Hearing Care Professionals.

During that time, I had the privilege of helping thousands of people navigate their hearing loss journey—from their first hearing test through the inevitable adjustments, troubleshooting sessions, and breakthrough moments when everything finally clicks.

While I no longer work in the field, those years gave me deep insight into both the technical and deeply personal sides of hearing loss. I witnessed the frustration of trying to follow conversations at family dinners, the embarrassment of asking "what?" one too many times, and the genuine joy when someone hears their grandchild's voice clearly for the first time in years.

This book grew out of countless conversations with patients who felt overwhelmed by the process—people who were given excellent devices but not enough guidance on how to actually live with them. I watched too many people struggle with issues that could have been easily resolved if they'd just known what to expect or who to ask.

I wrote this guide as the resource I wish I could have given every person who walked into my office: honest, practical advice that covers not just the science and technology, but the emotional journey, the awkward moments, and the small victories that come with adjusting to hearing aids.

Consider this your welcome guide to a world that can feel confusing and technical, written by someone who's been there, listened to thousands of stories, and wants to make your journey a little easier and a lot less overwhelming.

Most importantly, I'm no longer selling anything—I'm simply sharing what I've learned in hopes that your path to better hearing is smoother than it might otherwise be.

Hearing Aid Glossary

Whether you're new to hearing aids or just need a refresher, here's a handy glossary of the most common terms, plus a list of trustworthy resources where you can learn more or get support.

Understanding Your Hearing

Audiogram – A chart that shows the softest sounds you can hear at various frequencies. Think of it as a map of your unique hearing pattern that helps your audiologist program your hearing aids.

Decibel (dB) – The unit used to measure how loud sounds are. Normal conversation is around 60 dB, while a lawnmower is about 90 dB.

Frequency – How high or low a sound is, measured in Hertz (Hz). Higher frequencies include sounds like birds chirping, while lower frequencies include sounds like a bass drum.

Types of Hearing Loss

Sensorineural Hearing Loss – Hearing loss caused by damage to the inner ear or auditory nerve. This is the most common type and is usually permanent, but hearing aids can help significantly.

Conductive Hearing Loss – Hearing loss caused by problems in the outer or middle ear that block sound from reaching the inner ear. This type can sometimes be treated medically.

Hearing Aid Styles

Behind-the-Ear (BTE) – A hearing aid style where the main body sits behind your ear, connected to an earmold or dome in your ear canal.

In-the-Ear (ITE) – A hearing aid style that fits directly in your outer ear. These are custom-made to fit your ear shape.

Receiver-in-Canal (RIC) – A popular style where the receiver (speaker) sits in your ear canal while the main body sits behind your ear.

Hearing Aid Components

Microphone – The component that picks up sound from your environment. Most modern hearing aids have multiple microphones.

Amplifier – The processor inside the hearing aid that adjusts sound based on your specific hearing loss pattern.

Receiver – The part of the hearing aid that sends sound into your ear canal (essentially a tiny speaker).

Directional Microphone – A microphone that focuses on sound in front of you to help with speech understanding, especially in noisy environments.

Hearing Aid Accessories

Dome – A soft, replaceable silicone tip that fits in your ear canal on receiver-in-canal hearing aids. These come in different sizes and styles.

Earmold – A custom-molded piece made from an impression of your ear that helps hold the hearing aid in place and direct sound into your ear canal.

Wax Guard – A tiny filter that helps protect the hearing aid's receiver from earwax and debris. These need regular replacement.

Common Issues & Solutions

Feedback – A high-pitched whistling sound caused by amplified sound looping back into the hearing aid microphone. This usually happens when hearing aids don't fit properly, when there's wax buildup, or when you cup your hand near your ear.

Occlusion Effect – The strange, hollow sound of your own voice when an earmold or dome blocks your ear canal. This typically improves as you adjust to your hearing aids over the first few weeks.

Adjustment Period – The time it takes to get comfortable with new hearing aids, usually 2-4 weeks. Your brain needs time to relearn how to process sounds you may not have heard clearly in years.

Modern Features

Streaming – Sending audio (like phone calls, music, or TV) directly from a Bluetooth-enabled device to your hearing aids. Most newer hearing aids offer this feature.

Telecoil – A small coil that picks up magnetic signals from hearing loop systems in theaters, churches, and other public venues.

Remember: Getting used to hearing aids is a process. Be patient with yourself, and don't hesitate to contact your audiologist if you have questions or need adjustments.

Troubleshooting Quick-Reference

Common Hearing Aid Issues & How to Handle Them

Problem: No Sound at All

Check These First:

- Dead or incorrectly inserted battery
- Device switched off
- Wax blockage in tip, dome, or tubing
- Volume set too low

Quick Fixes:

1. Replace battery or recharge device completely
2. Verify hearing aid is switched on (check power button/switch)
3. Inspect for wax buildup and clean tip, dome, or tubing
4. Increase volume using device controls or smartphone app

Problem: Weak or Distorted Sound

Common Causes:

- Low battery power
- Microphone blocked by debris or moisture
- Recent moisture exposure

Try This:

1. Replace battery or fully recharge device
2. Gently brush microphone port with soft, dry brush
3. Use hearing aid drying kit or dehumidifier overnight
4. Check for loose connections in tubing (BTE models)

Problem: Whistling or Feedback

Why This Happens:

- Improper fit allowing sound to leak out
- Volume setting too high
- Earwax buildup creating poor seal

Solutions:

1. Remove and carefully reinsert hearing aid for proper fit
2. Lower volume slightly using controls or app
3. Schedule professional ear cleaning if wax buildup suspected

4. Try different dome size for better seal (consult provider first)

Problem: Intermittent Sound (Cutting In/Out)

Likely Culprits:

- Dirty or corroded battery contacts
- Moisture affecting internal electronics
- Loose wiring connections

Fix Attempts:

1. Open battery door and gently clean contacts with soft, dry brush
2. Use hearing aid dryer or dehumidifier for 6-8 hours
3. Check all connections and tubing for secure fit
4. Try fresh battery to rule out power issues

Problem: Won't Connect to Smartphone App

Connection Issues:

- Bluetooth disabled on phone
- Outdated app version
- Previous pairing conflict

Reconnection Steps:

1. Enable Bluetooth in phone settings

2. Update hearing aid app through app store

3. "Forget" device in Bluetooth settings, then re-pair

4. Follow manufacturer's pairing instructions exactly

5. Restart both devices if connection still fails

Problem: Uncomfortable Fit

Comfort Concerns:

- Wrong dome/tip size or style
- Incorrect insertion technique
- Tubing too long/short (BTE models)
- Ear canal changes over time

Comfort Solutions:

1. Try different dome/tip size (smaller or larger)

2. Practice proper insertion technique with mirror

3. Schedule fitting adjustment with hearing care provider

4. Ask about different dome materials if irritation persists

When to Call Your Provider

Contact your hearing care professional immediately if:

- Multiple troubleshooting attempts fail

- Physical damage to device is visible

- Unusual sounds, smells, or sensations occur

- Discomfort persists despite fit adjustments

- Device is still under warranty and having issues

Before You Call:

- Note specific symptoms and when they occur

- Try basic troubleshooting steps listed above

- Have your device model and serial number ready

- Mention any recent changes (new medications, ear infections, etc.)

Prevention Tips

Daily Maintenance:

- Clean devices every evening with provided tools

- Store in protective case or drying kit overnight

- Check battery levels regularly

- Handle with clean, dry hands

Weekly Care:

- Deep clean with manufacturer-approved wipes

- Inspect tubing and domes for wear or damage

- Test all functions including volume and program settings

Remember: Most hearing aid issues are simple fixes. When in doubt, gentle cleaning and fresh batteries solve many common problems!

Resources

Resources

- **Hearing Loss Association of America (HLAA)** – www.hearingloss.org Great for peer support, advocacy, and news on hearing loss topics.

- **BetterHearing.org (Better Hearing Institute)** – **https://www.betterhearing.org/** Consumer-focused information and hearing loss simulator tools

- **Hearing Health Foundation** - https://hearinghealthfoundation.org/ Research updates and tinnitus resources

- **AARP Hearing Center** - https://www.aarphearingsolutions.com/ Practical advice, insurance guidance

- **Consumer Reports Hearing Aid Reviews** - https://www.consumerreports.org/health/hearing-aids/ Independent product testing and buying guides

- **American Speech-Language-Hearing Association (ASHA)** – www.asha.org Offers professional information on audiology, hearing loss, and related services.

- **National Institute on Deafness and Other Communication Disorders (NIDCD)** – www.nidcd.nih.gov Government-funded site with research-based information.

- **Your Audiologist or Hearing Specialist** Don't underestimate the value of one-on-one support. Ask questions. Request follow-ups. Share your wins and challenges—they're there to help.

Thank You

Thank you for taking the time to read *The Hearing Aid Handbook*. I hope it brought you clarity, comfort, and confidence as you navigate the world of hearing aids.

If this book helped you—or someone you care about—I'd be truly grateful if you left a quick review on Amazon. Your feedback not only helps other readers find this book, but it also helps me continue sharing useful, honest guidance.

To learn more, get in touch, or discover upcoming releases, visit:

www.SideBPublishing.com

Your journey matters. Thanks for letting me be part of it.

—David L. Etheridge

www.ingramcontent.com/pod-product-compliance
Lightning Source LLC
Chambersburg PA
CBHW020607030426
42337CB00013B/1249